HOW TO ACHIEVE THE BEST STRENGHT TRAINING

Maria Ann

Table of Contents

INTRODUCTION

Strength or resistance training includes physical exercise aimed at improving strength and endurance. Often associated with lifting weights. It can also include various training techniques such as calisthenics, isometrics and plyometrics.

When done properly, strength training is associated with increased muscle, tendon, ligament and bone strength and toughness, improved joint function, reduced injury risk, increased bone density, increased metabolism, fitness, and an improved heart. Functional training generally employs techniques to gradually increase muscle power output through progressive weight gain and uses a variety of exercises and types of equipment that target specific muscle groups. Although it is anaerobic, some proponents have adapted it to provide the benefits of aerobic exercise through circuit training. Strength training typically produces lactic acid within the muscle, which is a limiting factor in exercise performance. Regular endurance training leads to skeletal muscle adaptations that can prevent lactate levels from rising during strength training.

Many sports and physical activities focus on strength training or use it as part of their training regimen.

CHAPTER ONE

WARMING UP

When life gets hectic and you're incredibly busy (so, all day, every day), it's tempting to start working out to maximize the time you have. But when you skip the warm-up and just go from 0 to 60, you're setting up your body less efficiently and you run the risk of injury.

Exercising without a warm-up is a big no-no, during exercise your muscles get shorter and longer, and if they're not warmed up or "prepared" your muscles are very vulnerable. torn and stretched. The key elements of a warm-up are increasing core body temperature, mobility, muscle activation, and building technique. "By increasing body temperature, you relax the tissues around joints, increasing their range of motion. Better flexibility does two things: allows your body to move better through the movements. exercise and help protect you from injury. "Incorporating movement will help reduce the risk of injury and help the body use the correct muscles for certain movements and prepare them for energy production. The strengthening section includes a warm-up of the body. For example, you can Warm up with a squat to prepare your body for the squat later in the actual workout.

So what can a time pressed individuals do? The truth is that you really only need five minutes to warm up. You just have to stop seeing it as a waste of time for your workout, and realize instead that it helps you to better maximize the minimal time you have.

A good warm-up should be specific to the range of motion you need for that particular exercise. So if you're going to do an upper body lift, you may want to spend more time prepping your shoulders and thoracic spine (upper back) and activating your glutes and glutes. On the other hand, if you're about to run or sprint, you may want to raise your hips and ankles as well as activate your glutes. "

There are many warm-ups you can do, to set up a great 5-minute warm-up that you can use before most weight training sessions. Experts also recommend foam rolling before doing this move to help release any existing tension or soreness in the muscles.

Here's a quick rundown of the startup process:

- 8 hip inward rotations, 8 hip outward rotations (each side)
- 8 front arm circles, 8 back arm circles
- 2 minutes skipping rope
- 8 outputs
- 12 deep inversions to lift the knee
- 15 squats with 10 reps at the end

And here's how to do each exercise:

Hip circle - 8 sets,

Hip rotations are a great way to relax the hips. If your hips are tight, they're important in helping you prepare for lower body exercises. Tight hips can prevent the surrounding muscles from pulling properly, especially the muscles, which can lead to compensation and tension in other parts of the body.

Raise one knee to 90 degrees. Cross your hips, forming a circle as big as your knees. Make the movement as wide as possible while remaining steady.

Continue to rotate slowly for eight reps, then change direction for eight reps. Repeat with the other leg.

Arm circle - forward 8 times, back 8 times

Arm circles are a great (and super easy) way to release tension in the shoulders and warm up the joints,

Stand with your feet shoulder-width apart, with your hands flat. • Slowly swing your arms forward in a circular motion. You will feel your shoulders relax as you walk.

Continue the circular motion for eight repetitions. Then, circle the arms in the opposite direction for eight moves.

Jump rope - 2 minutes

Jumping rope is one of the fastest ways to get your heart rate up and warm up. Jumping for two minutes at a moderate pace will do the trick. You will feel your heart beat faster. Don't be afraid to be fancy.

if you are comfortable with the rope. Bonus: jumping rope is also a great warm-up for your arms and shoulders!

• Rope and jump for 2 minutes. Output - 8 repetitions

Escapes are especially good for stretching your hamstrings and also activating your core. With this move, you will practice flexibility, mobility and strength. Speed up to increase your heart rate even more.

Start with your feet hip-width apart, hands at your sides.

Bend at your hips to keep your hands on the ground; crawl into a high plank position. • Pause for a few seconds with your shoulders on your wrists and your abs.

Crawling hands to feet and standing up.

Do eight repetitions.

Reverse Lunge to Knee Raise - 12 reps on each side

The lungs work the glutes, glutes, and hamstrings. Also, going straight from lunge to lift requires some serious core strength and stability.

Stand with feet hip-width apart.

Take a long step back with your right foot. Bend both knees as you lower yourself until your right knee is about 6 inches off the ground. • Push your right leg to stand up and bring your knee forward at a 90-degree angle.

Immediately step your right foot back into another inversion.

Do 12 reps for one leg, then 12 for the other leg.

Squats - 15 reps

Squats help you build glutes, glutes, and hamstrings. And depending on the form of strength training you do, chances are you'll do the squat at some point, with or without weights. Doing a few moves as part of a warm-up helps your body get used to the movement before progressing.

Stand with feet shoulder width apart, toes slightly apart, hands in front of chest.

Bend knees and hips to squat, bringing buttocks to knee level. Keep your chest high.

Walk on your heels to return to standing position. Do 15 repetitions.

Squat Pulses - 10 seconds

After performing 15 squats, squat for 10 seconds. It works the muscles in a slightly different way, and the extra speed increases your heart rate a bit too. Remember to keep your back flat (not arched or rounded) and chest up.

INTENTIONTALLY LEFT BLANK

CHAPTER TWO

PRINCIPLE FOR A GREAT TRAINING

As trainers and fitness professionals, it's essential to remember that every client and member we work with begins their strength training journey with a different background and understanding of the principles of strength training. Strength training and strength best practices. Many people don't know the science behind strength training.

- This lack of deeper understanding increases the importance of integrating education into new employee training, customer training, and conversing with members. Whether we are working with a seasoned exerciser who is already well versed in strength training or with a brand new client, it is essential to assess knowledge. their basics and incorporate instructional tips that will help advance their knowledge and beyond. their progress. The main educational topics to include in these conversations are the following principles of strength
    - overload
    - Progress
    - specificity
    - Rest and recovery
    - Nutrition and hydration

SIZE WEIGHT AND OVER LIGHT

Newbies to bodybuilding must know when to increase the weights their clients use and how to progress over time. It is important to educate about the importance of observation in making these assessments. For example, a person should observe that they do not feel fatigued at the end of exercises with proper form (and can easily do 5-6 more reps) or if they do not feel challenged. by exercise habits.

When educating our clients, it is important to explain that this observation may mean they are not using the most appropriate weight size and incorporate the fitness principle of progressive overload into the same. this explanation.

The fitness principle of progressive overload states that we must overload our neuromuscular systems over time to create and maintain physiological adaptations from strength training. On that same note, it's important to educate that when we strength train, we break down muscle fibres and try to overload this system to build them back stronger.

Keeping this goal in mind is the reason why you feel tired from the last rep of a certain set of exercises (with proper form), to be able to move less weight and perform less. more representative at the end of the session.

It's best if you inform your new workout clients that when they use the right weight size and challenge themselves during their workouts, they may not be able to train with intensity. same or use the same fee they started with. with the beginning of the exercise session. Overloading the neuromuscular system over time with the right weight size helps the body adapt and build back stronger.

principle of progress

Educating about progress is important. This indicates that no training time, distance traveled, or weight used in a particular exercise or activity should progress beyond her 10 weeks. Adhering to the 10% rule allows your body to gradually adapt and reduces the chance of overuse injuries.

When I encourage my clients and members to train with this 10% rule, I tell them that they shouldn't be afraid to lift heavier weights. However, explain that it is important not to sacrifice good exercise form for weight gain. Form is more important than speed or stress. If you're not sure if the 10% price increase is necessary, it's helpful to let the client know that they should start with a 5% price increase and re-evaluate from there.

Another helpful tip for new lifters is what to do if your weight size is in-between for a particular exercise. People new to strength training don't realize that if they get too tired in the middle of a set to continue with more reps, they can quickly grab a lighter weight and do the final reps.

This will give you an extra benefit towards your strength and endurance goals. Ultimately, applying this tip as needed will help these individuals become stronger and complete full sets with heavier loads. Educational tips like this may seem obvious to fitness professionals, but they can make a big difference for someone new to strength training.

Principle of specificity

Another important principle that customers need to be educated on is the principle of specificity. The fitness principle of specificity states that adjustments or changes in body strength are specific to the type of exercise. In other words, individuals only improve in their behavioural and practice skills. As far as strength training is concerned, it can be explained by individuals improving their training content.

We would like to share some frequently asked questions from our members and customers when talking about the specificity principle. The answer is often to practice and do more push-ups. Infact, incorporating other chest exercises can increase your overall muscle endurance and strength.

But in order to get better at a particular movement pattern or movement, that movement pattern or movement needs to be practiced and improved. For example, if a person wants to get better and adjust their body to run more, I have to run.

Fitness professionals need to educate those new to strength training not to skip or eliminate things that may be difficult for them. What is difficult for a person can be a clear sign that it is what they need most to become strong.

As fitness professionals, it's important to educate them about the importance of doing exactly what they want to do in order to improve their strength training. convey the importance of

rest and relaxation

Our muscles have an ideal training time-length-tension ratio. Muscles that are too long and overstretched, too tight or too strong can lead to physical pain and injury.

That's why it's important to incorporate active recovery techniques, training, and rest days, like active and passive flexibility, into a strength and fitness program. weekly. As fitness professionals, educating new members and clients about the importance of rest and recovery is essential to achieving their goals.

Make sure to educate on the topic to help reduce overuse and unnecessary overuse injuries. Let new clients know that rest and recovery is where most of the physiological adaptation occurs from strength training and is often the missing link in many fitness programs. The relationship between rest and progress, lack of rest, and possible injury risk needs to be explained before it's too late. On the topic of rest and recovery, let's share what it means to rest and recover beyond passive static stretching, range-of-motion exercises, and foam rolling exercises. Rest and recovery also mean getting enough sleep and incorporating proper nutrition. Adequate rest of 7-9 hours per night is essential to aid in the recovery process.

Additionally, taking a day off from strength training, using self-liberation, and weekly prioritizing active movement and passive stretching are all important steps. In addition to sleep hygiene and wellness regeneration strategies, it is important to educate members and clients about the importance of nutrition and hydration when starting or improving a strength training program.

NUTRITION HYDRATION

As a fitness professional, I recommend promoting nutrition and hydration strategies that will help all individuals (not just athletes) function well in their daily lives and in the process. train their strength.

It is essential to educate new clients about hydration needs before, during, and after training. There are strategies to help make these recommendations very specific to an individual. However, as a guide, you should drink at least 20 ounces about 60-90 minutes before a workout, about 4-6

1 oz (4-6 puffs) every 15 minutes during exercise and approximately 16-24 oz post-exercise.

Regarding nutrition, it is important to educate members about the importance of pre-workout and post-workout fuel. It's the fitness expert's job to communicate the importance of a healthy diet to her at least two hours before training.

Also, explain how eating a healthy snack about 30 minutes before strength training can help if you haven't had a proper meal. In addition to pre-workout, talk about what you need to do post-workout so you can start the recovery process. As a rule of thumb, tell new clients to eat a healthy snack (containing lean protein and complex carbs) within 30-45 minutes after their workout. You also need to make them realize that the sooner you do this, the better it is for your body and your recovery.

It helps me understand the "why" behind all this information. How consuming enough protein supports tissue repair, and how consuming enough of the right types of carbohydrates can help maximize the recovery process and replenish energy stores.

CHAPTER THREE

TYPES

The basic principle of strength training is to use weight and force through a series of repetitive movements to create changes in strength, endurance, and size by overloading muscle groups. Strength training usually involves using weight machines or lifting free weights at the gym, but you can also use your own body weight and resistance bands. Fitness equipment supports your body, makes sure you are in the right position when lifting, allows for good form, and helps isolate muscle groups. I need to think more deeply about things and I can understand my body better.

There are four different techniques that weights can be used to build key aspects of strength. The main difference between techniques is the number of times you do each exercise (reps) and how many times you complete a series of reps (called sets).

Beginners should start with light weights. It's important to fully master technique and form before challenging your muscles with weight gain.

Here four different types of strength training are:

1. Strength training for strength

This technique aims to improve the explosive power of the muscles. This workout increases your ability to perform powerful movements in a short amount of time. For example, jump or start a fast sprint. This type of training is often used to improve athletic performance. This type of training uses "fast-twitch fibres (which produce more power and power than "slow-twitch fibres), but fatigues much faster and takes longer to recover.

2. Strength training for strength

This type of training is designed to achieve maximum strength and size. H. Ability to lift and push heavy objects. Powerlifters build strength and bodybuilders build muscle mass. The larger the muscle fibre the more force you can exert.

3. Strength training for muscle hypertrophy

This technique is especially useful for weight loss as it helps achieve a toned appearance and builds muscle mass in the body. it also helps reduce age-related muscle wasting that can lead to weakness. increase.

4. Strength training for muscle endurance

fast-twitch fibres are the largest and strongest muscle fibres in the body, and the more you exercise, the more you utilize them. However, when you do muscle endurance training, slow twitch fibres work and you can perform movements like rowing for a long time. Your body recruits muscle fibres based on the strength demands placed on it. Therefore, in muscle endurance sports, strength training focuses on the lower intensity demands of building slow-twitch fibres.

CHAPTER FOUR

PHYSICAL BENEFITS

If there is anything you can do to improve your health, strength training should be at the top of your list. This involves him using one or more muscle groups to perform specific tasks. B. Lift weights or squat down. With growing evidence of its many benefits, strength training has become a fundamental part of most exercise programs. If you've ever thought about strength training, how can it benefit your life?.

- make you stronger

Having stronger muscles will make it much easier to perform everyday tasks such as Carrying heavy groceries or walking around with children.

Additionally, it helps improve athletic performance in sports that require speed, power and power, and may even support endurance athletes by maintaining lean muscle mass.

- Burn Calories Efficiently

Strength training can help boost your metabolism in two ways. First, building muscle increases your metabolic rate. Muscle is more metabolically efficient than fat, so you can burn more calories at rest.

- and losing fat will make you look slimmer.

-

- Gaining muscle and losing fat will make you look slimmer.

This is because muscle is denser than fat. So even if you don't see any change in the numbers on the scale, you can lose inches from your waistline.

Also, when you lose body fat and build stronger and bigger muscles, your muscles become more defined and look stronger and leaner.

- Reduces the risk of fall

Strength training reduces the risk of falls because the body can be better supported.

Fortunately, many forms of strength training have been found to be beneficial, including Tai Chi, strength training, resistance bands, bodyweight exercises.

- Boost your self esteem

Strength training can significantly boost your confidence. It helps you overcome challenges, work toward your goals, and appreciate the strength of your body. In particular, it can increase your self-efficacy (the belief that you can or can complete a task), which can greatly increase your self-confidence.

- Increased mobility

Contrary to popular belief, strength training improves flexibility.

Strength training increases joint mobility (ROM) and improves mobility and flexibility. Also, people with weak muscles tend to have low ROM and flexibility.

For best results, make sure you are running the full ROM of the exercise. In other words, use the full range of motion around your joints. For example, squat as much as you can without sacrificing your form.

INTENTIONTALLY LEFT BLANK

CHAPTER FIVE

MENTAL BENEFIT

- Reduces abdominal fat

Fat stored around the abdomen, especially visceral fat, is associated with an increased risk of chronic diseases such as heart disease, non-alcoholic fatty liver disease, type 2 diabetes and certain types of cancer.

The benefit of strength training is to reduce belly and overall body fat.

- Reduces blood pressure

Regular weight training lowers blood pressure, lowers total and LDL (bad) cholesterol, and improves circulation by strengthening the heart and blood vessels.

Strength training also helps you maintain a healthy weight and control blood sugar levels. High blood sugar is an important risk factor for heart disease.

- Helps control blood sugar levels

Strength training reduces the risk of developing diabetes and helps those affected to better manage their diabetes.

Skeletal muscle helps increase insulin sensitivity. It also lowers blood sugar levels by removing glucose from the blood and sending it to muscle cells. As a result, increased muscle mass helps improve blood sugar control.

- Reduces the risk of cancer

Visceral fat not only increases the risk of heart disease and diabetes, but is also associated with an increased risk of cancer. Visceral fat cells produce high levels of a cancer-causing protein called fibroblast growth factor-2 (FGF2).

- Lower the risk of injury

Incorporating strength training into your daily exercise routine can reduce your risk of injury. Strength training helps improve strength, range of motion, and flexibility in muscles, ligaments, and tendons. This provides added strength around major joints such as knees, hips and ankles, providing better protection against injuries.

Additionally, strength training helps compensate for muscle imbalances. For example, a stronger core, hamstrings, and glutes will make your lower back easier when you lift, reducing the risk of back injury.

Finally, adult and youth athletes who do strength training have a lower risk of injury.

- Prevention and management of osteoporosis

Powerful mineral density, weight-bearing exercise where standing and gravity presses against the body easily loads and strengthens bones and muscles.

Also, each time a muscle contracts, it pulls on the bone to which it is attached, stimulating the cells within the bone to produce structural proteins and transport minerals to the bone.

- Improves brain health

Strength training can improve brain performance throughout a person's lifetime, but the effects are probably greatest in older adults who suffer from cognitive decline. For example, men and women aged 55 to 86 with mild disabilities who did strength training twice a week for six months significantly improved their cognitive test scores. However, cognitive test scores decreased when participants spent stretching their workouts.

keeping in mind that high-intensity strength training increases the flow of blood, oxygen, and other nutrients throughout the body, including the brain, the key may be getting blood flow.

mental benefits

The benefits of strength training for you can be a personal and unique experience. Here are some common ways strength training can help your mental health. make me feel better

Strength training can improve your mood in many ways. Setting goals, developing habits, and following a routine can improve your mood. Plus, the endorphins released by strength training can boost feel-good chemicals that help you see the bright side of life.

Strength training can also reduce other depressive symptoms in many people. Of course, if you have symptoms of depression or other mental health issues, it's important to consult a mental health professional.

However, there is no downside to doing strength training or other physical activity to improve your symptoms. Talk to your doctor first to make sure the exercise you want to do is allowed.

The benefits of exercise, including strength training, to ameliorate certain mental illnesses, it is imperative that you seek treatment if you have symptoms. Never stop taking prescription drugs or other treatments without consulting your health care provider and discussing the problem first.

- Strengthens the mind-body connection

Strength training requires a high degree of mind-body connection due to the risks associated with using heavy weights. It's important to know how your body is responding.

When we listen to our body and move with intention to let our body guide us, such as how much weight to lift, which movements feel good and which ones don't. It tells us that the body is a reliable and wise leader.

However, keep in mind that strength training can also be done in a way that overrides the body's wisdom.

Having a no-frills, no-gain mentality, or following the signals your body may be sending while doing what your trainer tells you to do, can lead to misunderstandings, disconnections, and ultimately may lead to injury. Pay attention to how you are feeling and take the time to check on yourself to make sure you are not ignoring these signals.

- Reduce stress and anxiety

Strength training can reduce stress and anxiety by lowering the stress hormone cortisol. Additionally, lowering cortisol reduces anxiety.

When you do strength training, your mind releases endorphins, the body's "feel good" hormones, lowering cortisol levels and making you feel better after exercise.

Strength training, in particular, can reduce anxiety by up to 20% (for study participants). This may have increased their confidence in their own abilities and coping skills, leading to a sense of proficiency.

Improving skills is most likely to increase self-confidence and self-esteem and lead to reduced anxiety resolver. Biological changes in the muscles and brain work together to reduce anxiety symptoms, but more needs to be done to draw firm conclusions. Research is required.

- Strength training helps your body maintain hormonal health. Our hormones affect every part of our body, especially our emotions and mental state.

INTENTIONALLY LEFT BLANK

CHAPTER SIX

FOOD FOR OPTIMUM PERFORMANCE

food energy

The energy requirements of a strength trainer exceed those of the average person. It's not uncommon for male and female strength trainers, especially those still growing, to need in excess of 2400-3000 and 2200-2700 calories per day, respectively. The amount of energy a particular food contains depends on the food's macronutrient (carbohydrate, protein and fat) content.

Macronutrients > Energy Content

carbs > 4 Kcal/gram

Protein > 4 kcal/gram

Alcohol* > 7 kcal/g

Fat > 9 kcal/g

*While alcohol is not considered a macronutrient, it is important to realize that it is high in calories and can contribute to unwanted weight gain.

Carbohydrates serve as the primary source of energy during high-intensity activity. Healthy food sources of carbohydrates include fruits, vegetables, whole grains, breads and pasta.

Dietary fats also play an important role in helping individuals meet their energy needs and support healthy hormone levels. Healthy fat sources include nuts, nut butters, avocados, olives and coconut oil. I have. Limit the use of vegetable oils such as corn, cottonseed, and soybean oil.

Dietary protein plays an important role in muscle repair and growth. Preferred protein sources include lean meats, eggs, dairy products (yogurt, milk, cottage cheese), and legumes.

- Tips to Shine with the Right Diet

1. Plan to eat a variety of fruits and vegetables each day. Eat at least servings of fruit and vegetables daily. A serving is about the size of a baseball. Fruits and vegetables are packed with the energy and nutrients you need for training and regeneration. Also rich in antioxidants, these foods can help fight off illnesses such as colds and flu.

2. For a powerful source of energy, choose whole-grain carbohydrate sources such as whole-wheat bread, whole-wheat pasta, and high-fibre cereals. Limit refined grains and sugar, such as sweet cereals, white bread, and bagels. Get more benefits from whole grain products.

Choose healthy protein sources such as chicken, turkey, fish, peanut butter, eggs, nuts and legumes.

3. A 2% drop in hydration levels can negatively impact your performance, so stay hydrated with fluids. You can choose from milk, water, 100% fruit juice, and sports drinks. However, be aware that sports drinks and his 100% fruit juices tend to have higher total sugar levels, and in the case of fruit juices, many of the health benefits found in whole foods are lost. Also, be careful not to confuse sports drinks like Gatorade with "energy" drinks like Red Bull and similar drinks.

4. Stick to whole foods whenever possible, as opposed to highly processed foods.

- Planning a nutritious meal

Without getting enough calories from the healthiest food sources, you'll struggle to reach your performance goals. Plan a nutritious meal by choosing at least one food from each category.

Carbohydrates

· Fruit

· Oatmeal

· Starchy vegetables (sweet/white potatoes, squash)

· Non-starchy vegetables (broccoli, leafy greens)

· Whole-grain bread or crackers

· High-fibre, non-sugary cereals

Quinoa

· Brown or wild rice

Protein

· Whole eggs (white and yolk)

· Greek yogurt

· Milk

· String cheese

· Lean red meats

· Poultry

· Fish

· Hummus

Healthy fat

· Avocado

· Peanut butter

· Nuts and seeds

· Coconut oil

- Hydration

Adequate hydration is a key element in sports performance. Most athletes benefit from developing a personal hydration plan. A general rule for training is to consume a minimum:

· Two cups of fluid prior to training

· Four to six ounces of fluid every 15 minutes of exercise

Your post event/training hydration needs are impacted by your overall pre- to post-fluid losses. To properly assess this, weigh yourself immediately before and after your workout. Replace 16 ounces of fluid for every pound of weight lost. Optimal hydration includes water, skimmed milk, or 100% juice. Sports drinks are ideal for sports that require rapid hydration and electrolyte replacement.

CHAPTER SEVEN

FOODS TO AVOID FOR OPTIMUM PERFORMANCE

It is recommended to eat and prepare before going to the gym. However, choosing the wrong diet can make your workout more difficult and hinder your intended progress. It's going to end up.

Inadvertently eating or drinking before exercise or exercising on an empty stomach can damage the body's systems and cause cramps.

For the best workout, avoid her seven foods and drinks.

- linseed

Linseed is rich in fibre and is naturally good for the body. However, too much fibre can make your stomach bloated and bloated, interfering with your exercise routine. You should avoid consuming high-fibre foods two hours before and after exercise. Besides flaxseeds, do not add fibre, bran, vegetable salads or high-fibre baked foods.

- protein bar

Don't be fooled by supermarket protein bars. Many protein bars have over 200 calories, are very low in protein, and are basically the same as a chocolate bar. If the protein bar contains less than 10 grams of protein, it may lower blood sugar more quickly and make you feel tired faster. Pay attention to the nutrition table on the package. Choose a protein bar with 200 calories or less and a 1:1 sugar to protein ratio. fast food

A high-carb, high-protein meal isn't the same as the burgers and fries you get at your local fast food joint. Junk food is high in fat and takes at least 4 hours to fully digest.

When digesting food, the heart concentrates on pumping blood to the stomach to aid in the process. Blood flow to muscles is reduced and muscles have to absorb large amounts of blood during strenuous activities such as exercise. may collapse. Fast food is best avoided, but healthy high-fat snacks like cheese, avocados and almonds can also make you feel sluggish. why? The process of converting fat into energy is thought to be less efficient than carbohydrates and proteins. The complex process of fat digestion in the body can lead to stomach cramps and discomfort. Choose the simplest processed rice, pasta, potatoes, or meat possible. A good pre-workout nutrition guideline is a 4:1 carbohydrate to protein ratio for maximum energy.

- dairy products

Even low-fat milk, which is said to be a diet food, can have adverse effects on the body during exercise. Protein is your primary source of energy and can help your muscles recover, but high-protein foods and drinks don't contain enough carbohydrates, so they use up your energy more quickly. Since protein enters the blood slowly, even if you have just eaten a large meal, you will feel tired and shivering.

- sugar

Foods high in simple carbohydrates and sugar, including healthy smoothies, provide only temporary energy, not the sustained energy needed for training. You need the help of the good bacteria that live within you. Consuming too many artificial sweeteners threatens the growth of good bacteria and interferes with nutrient absorption.

High-carb, sugary snacks can raise blood sugar levels and even cause you to pass out during a workout. it is best to avoid orange juice, isotonic drinks, sodas, and energy drinks when planning strenuous exercise. Caffeine can provide extra energy before exercise, but it can also mess up sleep patterns. Lack of sleep means you don't have enough energy for physical activity. Choose healthy espresso or tea over sodas and energy drinks. If you love smoothies, make your own at home with fresh fruit and protein powder.

- egg

Hard-boiled eggs are a good source of pure protein, but they don't have enough carbohydrates for balanced energy. Proteins and eggs also stay in your stomach longer before being digested, which makes you feel heavier during exercise. Also, eating raw eggs before exercising is not a good idea. Raw eggs contain Salmonella bacteria, which can cause abdominal pain and diarrhea. Instead of egg dishes, plain he is best replaced with yogurt or a mixture of cheese and fruit salad.

- Spicy food

Spicy food is good for nutrition because it allows you to burn calories faster, but this healthy value won't work if you eat spicy food before hitting the gym. Spicy foods can cause stomach pains and throat burns and interfere with your workout.

- green banana

Bananas are a good pre-workout snack, but make sure you choose yellow, ripe bananas. Choose bananas that do not have green spots that indicate they are unripe. The best way to tell if a banana is ripe is for brownish spots on the skin. At this ripeness, the sugar content in bananas makes them easier for the body to digest.

CHAPTER EIGHT

CONSEQUENCES OF LACK OF STRENGHT TRAINING

Most people agree that drunk driving, smoking, and sword swallowing are inherently risky activities. Surprisingly, sometimes doing nothing - not moving a muscle - can be life-threatening.

Not exercising, or even not engaging in physical activity, is a confirmed risk factor for early death. In fact, inactivity and a sedentary lifestyle cause more deaths worldwide than smoking or diabetes, according to a study published in the journal The Lancet. The researchers found that the least fit people (as determined by the treadmill test) had a 500% increased risk of premature death. first

- Getting a good night's sleep can be difficult.

Not getting enough sleep or tossing around at night doesn't seem to be a cause for concern. But if it happens regularly, it can lead to a host of health problems, from weight gain to diabetes to heart disease, poor immunity, mood swings and even accidents. So, poor sleep due to lack of physical activity can be life-threatening. Now consider the flip side: Have you ever fallen into the deepest, most satisfying, and most rejuvenating sleep after spending three hours in the fresh air working in the yard, kayaking, backpacking 10 miles? Or run a long distance race? Vigorous exercise, especially when done outdoors, is a very effective non-drug sleep aid, which you would overlook if you didn't exercise regularly.

- You may have high blood pressure.

Exercise helps your heart pump blood more efficiently. If your heart is fit, it will have to work less to pump blood and the force in your arteries will decrease. If you don't exercise, over time your cardiovascular fitness (CRF) will decrease. You will be more likely to have heart disease.

Even if you don't have any of the classic risk factors for heart disease, like high blood pressure, high cholesterol and obesity, being inactive can still lead to heart disease, which affects 6 million American.

- Your memory can fail more easily.

Scientists believe that exercise promotes neuroplasticity, the brain's ability to form new neural connections and adapt throughout life.

one area of this development is in the hippocampus, which governs memory and executive functions.

- Your blood sugar will go out of control.

Physical activity plays an important role in how your body processes carbohydrates, and even missing a few sessions can impair blood sugar control, according to a recent study published in the journal Diabetes. solstice. Even in the short term, reducing daily activity and stopping regular exercise cause the acute body changes associated with diabetes that can precede weight gain and obesity development.

Conversely, even a bout of moderate exercise can improve the way the body regulates blood sugar. You don't have to be an athlete to reap the benefits of exercise. seven

- You may increase your risk of certain cancers.

Does sitting all day increase cancer risk? It has not been scientifically proven, but sedentary behaviour is a risk factor for many chronic diseases and premature death. Although no studies have proven that lack of exercise causes cancer, numerous self-reported observational studies have provided evidence linking higher physical activity to a lower risk of cancer,

- Your knees and shoulders may be sore.

Joint pain can be caused by osteoarthritis, injury, repetitive motion at work, and aging, but inactivity is also a common cause of joint pain. Restricting your movement can weaken your muscles, worsen joint problems, and affect your posture, causing a host of other problems.

- Your “good” HDL cholesterol will drop.

Regular aerobic exercise is one of the most effective ways to increase high-density lipoprotein (HDL) cholesterol, known as good cholesterol. HDL cholesterol helps remove harmful cholesterol from your blood and is associated with a reduced risk of heart disease. If you don't exercise regularly and with enough intensity to raise your heart rate, your HDL will likely drop and your LDL (bad) cholesterol will increase. These activities are enough to speed up your heart rate and make it difficult for you to breathe. It's generally good for your HDL cholesterol, as well as LDL and triglycerides. Supplement this substance with a healthy diet

- Your bones may become brittle.

As you age, calcium from your bones is reabsorbed into your bloodstream. This causes a decrease in bone mass and can lead to brittle bones, a condition known as osteoporosis. Exercise is one of the main ways to prevent this bone loss. If you don't eat a lot, you increase your risk of age-related bone weakness. Resistance training with weights is recommended to increase bone density.

www.ingramcontent.com/pod-product-compliance
Lightning Source LLC
LaVergne TN
LVHW020533160826
845677LV00015B/4027
* 9 7 9 8 3 5 1 7 2 7 6 2 2 *